The Perfect Gift

Geraldine Naughton

Order this book online at www.trafford.com
or email orders@trafford.com

Most Trafford titles are also available at major online book retailers.

Printed in Victoria, BC, Canada.

ISBN: 978-1-4269-3411-7 (soft)
ISBN: 978-1-4269-3459-9 (ebook)

*Our mission is to efficiently provide the world's finest, most comprehensive book publishing
service, enabling every author to experience success. To find out how to publish your book, your
way, and have it available worldwide, visit us online at www.trafford.com*

Trafford rev. 5/27/2010

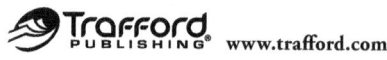 **www.trafford.com**

North America & international
toll-free: 1 888 232 4444 (USA & Canada)
phone: 250 383 6864 ♦ fax: 812 355 4082

AUTHOR: GERALDINE NAUGHTON

Geraldine has published three children's books, A WHALE
OF A TALE IN RIO-VISTA , THE LITTLE FISH and THE RAINY
DAY. She loves to envision and write stories that come to life
in colorful books for children of all ages to enjoy.

My book, THE PERFECT GIFT, is a story of true love and inspiration of two people who loved and cared so much for one another that they placed themselves second to the other in their everyday lives. Larry and Mollie were married for twenty nine years. Mollie battled cancer for four years and her biggest supporter and caregiver was her husband Larry. Unknown to everyone, Larry became ill, kept it a secret to himself and sacrificed his chances of treatment to enable him to take care of Mollie. Because of this sacrifice, Larry passed while Mollie continued to fight her battle with cancer with the help and support of her family.

I dedicate my book The Perfect Gift to my sister Mollie and her husband Larry and those whos lives had an impact from cancer.

To the family of cancer victims and surviors my hopes is that The Perfect Gift will give you some comfort in coping with this ungodly disease.

On July 5th, 1980, Mary Alice Naughton, known to everyone as Mollie, and Larry Moraski united in Marriage and a strong love grew for one another that cancer itself could not come between them.

Mollie walked down the aisle with our oldest brother Frank-o who took the place of our father who had passed away years earlier. Smiling beautifully, she walked down the aisle, making the most beautiful bride. She was a happy bride, and she wanted everyone to know just how happy she was. What better way to display her feelings than to smile radiantly. As she reached the altar arm in arm with Larry, the first words the priest spoke were, "Mollie you have the most beautiful smile." This is what I remember most about her wedding day, because it was so true.

Before their marriage they had purchased an older home at 110 Ash Street, Scranton, Pennsylvania. As the years went by, they would remodel it to their own liking.

Larry and Mollie where blessed with two sons. Their first son was born on May 26, 1982. They baptized him as Robert-named after an infant brother of Larry who had died shortly after birth.

Their second son, Danny was born on May 8th, 1984. Throughout the years, Mollie and Larry would be involved in many sports and drama activities with their sons. Their lives were no different than any other average family.

On Halloween they would fix their home up as a haunted house. Their nieces and nephews were so scared that they would cry because they had to go in. Larry would be Jason from Friday the 13th movie and his brother Steve would be Michael Meyers from the movie Halloween; both would play their roles to the fullest, and any kid including some adults would be scared to death to enter the Moraski's haunted house.

In December of 2005, their lives took a drastic turn. Mollie was diagnosed with advanced ovarian cancer. The doctors had scheduled her for surgery in January of 2006. During the surgery the doctors were hit with a surprise: not only did she have ovarian cancer, but Mollie had advanced uterine cancer as well. The doctors performed a complete hysterectomy which was followed with chemo and radiation to make sure all the cancer was gone.

Mollie made frequent trips to Allentown, for chemo treatments, hoping the cancer would never return. The chemo treatments took their toll on Mollie, making her very week and ill.

Throughout her treatments, Mollie spent a lot of time in the hospital because of the toll it took on her body and her organs. Finally the treatments were over. Three and one half years went by with no signs of cancer. Everyone thought she was going to beat it. Mollie was so happy with the thoughts of being cancer free that she decided to get a tattoo. Across her entire back was a tattoo of her Doctor, her husband Larry and herself with the words, "thank you for saving my life." When she proudly showed me her tattoo, I said, "My God Mollie didn't that hurt?" Her response was "Ger, after what I went through with my cancer and chemo, nothing hurts."

Unfortunately in November of 2008, Mollie started showing signs of the cancer returning.

She went to see her family doctor, Dr. McKenna, for a consultation and more tests. The tests showed small nodules throughout various parts of her body. With these findings, Dr. McKenna ordered more chemo treatments which Mollie would begin in December. During this time, I flew back to

Scranton to help with taking care of Mollie which would enable my two sisters, Nancy and Judy, and her husband Larry to have a break from the constant care she required. The night before I was to accompany Mollie to her first chemo treatment, she became upset, crying, "Why can't I remember anything? What's wrong with me that you're not telling me?"

It was all Larry, Judy and I could do to hold back our tears. "Mollie," I said, "we're not hiding anything from you. Tomorrow you will go for your first treatment, and we'll find out what's going on with you."

Mollie was so upset that night I had to sit and talk with her before she went to sleep. I reassured her we weren't hiding anything from her, and we would find out what we needed to know the next day at her chemo treatment.

After Mollie had fallen asleep, Larry and I went out on the porch. I cried to Larry how I felt that the cancer may have gone to her brain. She was so very confused and couldn't remember who called on the phone, or for that matter, if anyone had called including her husband. He looked at me and said, "I know, Ger, but I don't say anything, because if it is, there is nothing we could do about it."

I explained to Larry how Mollie had confided in me as to how she was afraid to die, and how I felt she had to find peace with herself. "Larry," I said, "I know in my heart she's not going to beat it this time, and she knows it too."

Larry looked at me and said, "You know Ger, with hesitation, I... I just don't say anything." We went back inside on that cold night, and I sat in a chair very quietly with a light on and began to write—this is what I do when I'm upset or at ends with myself. I began to write a poem of encouragement for Mollie, hoping it would help her to keep fighting this ungodly disease.

The next day I accompanied her to her first chemo treatment at the Mercy Hospital chemo center. It was then that we learned Mollie's medicine had been labeled wrong, and unknowingly, Larry had been giving her too much medicine.

This is what was making her confused, tired and at times incoherent. It was a great relief to all of us, because now we knew what was going on with Mollie, and that it wasn't the cancer going into her brain. After we got home and settled down for the evening, I gave Mollie the poem I had written for her. She read it, and then gave it to Larry to read. Mollie cried as she thanked me and of course Larry thought it was "so nice."

OUR MOLLIE

To my sister, Mollie, with a beautiful smile.

I know you've been ill for quite awhile.

I'm hoping to encourage you to continue to fight.

With my words of love I write for you tonight.

When life throws you a curve, just step aside.

Take one step forward, don't try to hide.

Your strength is of plenty, your courage might

Whatever life throws you, get ready to fight.

There's no hurdle you can't jump, no road you can't take.

To get to your destiny, your future, your faith.

When your thoughts are unhappy, don't let them get you down.

Just put on a smile and turn the frown upside down.

Your place in this world is wife, sister, and mother.

For you are "OUR MOLLIE" and there could be no other.

We love you Mollie.

December 12, 2008

Love, Gerri

During this Christmas visit, I had learned firsthand the love and admiration my brother-in-law, Larry, had for my sister Mollie. During the day while he was at work, I tended to her needs and did the house chores. Her first statement to me was, "Ger, could you make it as easy for Larry as possible? Would you please do the laundry?"

I laughed and said, "That's why I'm here. I want him to go to work, and not have to worry about you or how you are doing, or what house work needs to be done when he gets home."

When Larry got home from work, if there was running around to do such as the store, he would not complain, he would just go and get it done. After that Mollie was his responsibility, and he let me know it.

One evening, Mollie said she had to go to the bathroom because she wasn't feeling well. Larry and I went with her as she glided along using her walker. As we got to the bathroom door, she cried," It's going to come out." I quickly ran into the bathroom and got the clothes hamper to put it front of her, thinking she had to throw up. She started crying, "No Ger, the other way." "Forget it," she said in despair, "it's too late."

I looked at Larry and told him I would go in the bathroom and take care of her. "No," he said, "I'm home. I'll do it. I'll take care of her."

At this point, Mollie was dealing with incontinence, and to my surprise, Larry informed me that he would take care of her—which he did. I remember sitting in their parlor that night thinking how much Larry loved and adored my sister. For him to go and do whatever needed to be done and take care of her personal needs when it would have been easier for him to let me do it, showed how much he cared about her. After it was over, the three of us laughed about me running to get the hamper and putting it in front of her thinking she needed to throw up. I said, "Leave it up to me; I thought she had to throw up." After that experience, when she said she was sick and needed the bathroom, I certainly didn't waste my time running for a hamper.

On many occasions Mollie and I sat and discussed her feelings about her illness. She knew she wasn't going to beat it this time. "Too much, Ger," she said. "It's in too many places. God's going to take me this time, and I'm not going to be anyone's sister, wife, mother, anything." She cried.

I comforted her best I could with a story of our family tree. I took a picture of our Mom and Dad and tapped it to the wall in her bedroom where she could see it. I told her, when she felt this way, to look at their picture and remember they would be with God waiting for her, because we are all God's children, and he doesn't want any of us to suffer. I explained to her how our Mom and Dad would be reaching out to her because she suffered long enough; it was time for their baby to rest.

This seemed to give her some comfort, because she would always fall asleep after she heard the story. As for me, I would ask myself do I really believe this or am I just trying to make her feel better, or for that matter, make myself feel better. I honestly wasn't sure at that point how I felt, or what I believed in as far as life and death went. I knew deep in my heart that our baby sister wasn't going to beat it this time. I didn't let her know that I felt this way. However, I also knew that she was quite aware of how I felt. She made me promise her that when her time came, I would be there to hold her hand. Mollie told me many times that she was afraid to die, and I promised her that I would be there.

Mollie had good days and bad days during my December visit. At one point, she managed to get the strength to do some Christmas decorating. Larry was so happy when he got home from work and saw the decorations. He remarked, "Ahhh that looks so nice." While helping Mollie decorate, we turned on her singing reindeer. It began singing, "Here Comes Santa Claus...." At this point, Mollie and I began singing and dancing to the musical reindeer as her son Danny took videos. It didn't last very long. Mollie became dizzy after the first verse, causing her to sit and sing while I danced around like a nut. This was definitely a good day, and one I'll never forget. Of course, being able to watch the video whenever I want is a blessing. I always say technology these days is the greatest as long as there isn't a major black out.

Christmas got closer, and visitors were more frequent. Everyone loved the decorations. My favorite time was when Mollie and I painted our own ornaments for family, and we made a cake for Larry's birthday. Of course, Mollie didn't bake the cake; she had no energy for that. However, she did put the icing on it. That was one of the funniest and saddest days. It was during this time she was on too much medicine, and we didn't know it yet. Mollie couldn't get the icing to spread on the cake so she asked me for the "wheels for the spatula." I couldn't help it. I had to laugh. Yet, at the same time I was sad. It took her awhile, but she managed to get it done.

When Larry came home from work, the cake was definitely a surprise to him; he didn't know it was his birthday. A few family members and their sons came over, and we sang happy birthday to him. Of course everyone had a good laugh, including Mollie when Larry told everyone he didn't know it was his birthday!

My two weeks in Scranton went by too quickly. It was time for me to catch a plane back to California. The morning I left, Larry left me a note thanking me for my help, and I, in return, left him a note thanking him for loving my sister so much.

I called my sister almost every day to check on her and see how she was doing.

One day in January 2009, Mollie called my cell phone while I was at work. I quickly answered it thinking something was not right. "Ger," she said, "I have something to tell you." I replied, "What is it? Are you ok?" "Yes, I'm ok. It's Larry. He has liver cancer."

I was in shock. I could not believe what she had just told me. Mollie couldn't tell me much except to say he was going for tests, and she would let me know the outcome when they found out the results. I kept in contact with Mollie and Larry, but when I would ask about his test results, they would just say that they still didn't know much. My feeling was that neither of them wanted to talk about it.

In March I received a phone call from my sister Judy informing me Larry was being admitted to a hospice as we spoke. I heard of *hospice* but I'd never had firsthand experience with one. I asked Judy about it and what it was like. She explained, "Ger, it's a good thing. Larry will be made as comfortable as possible and free of pain."

"How is Mollie?" I asked? Judy told me that Mollie didn't know yet. "Larry and his sister Nancy are going to call her and tell her everything when Larry got settled in.

Judy explained to me that Larry had known he had cancer for some time. He didn't tell anyone or receive any treatment because he wouldn't have been able to take care of Mollie. We ended our phone conversation; my heart felt heavy and I had so many questions—how, why...?

I called Mollie and told her how very sorry I was. All she could do was say, "I know Ger, I know." Feeling helpless and far away, I sent Larry a basket of fruit with a personal letter letting him know how very pleasant and full of admiration my Christmas visit had been. I told him how much I loved him for the love he had for my sister, and that I loved him for who he was. Later I was told how happy he was that I felt that way. There are times in our lives when we just have to tell people how we feel and this was one of them.

I kept in contact with Judy as to Larry's condition and how our sister Mollie was dealing with this ungodly situation. Mollie and both sides of the Naughton and Moraski families spent much time at the hospice with Larry. Mollie would do all she could to keep up her strength and be strong for him. The following Tuesday, March 24, 2009, I received a phone call from my sister—Larry had passed away. A few hours later, I got another phone call. Mollie was being admitted to the hospital; she was septic which meant that she had blood poisoning throughout her body. Mollie wasn't able to go to Larry's viewing or his funeral—she was too ill to make it. Mollie recovered from her illness and went back home.

In April, I went back to visit Mollie again and help tend to her needs. It was her birthday, and she was not doing well. She missed her soul-mate and she told me,"Ger, people think I'm strong, but I'm not. I know God is going to take me, and I'm scared." Again, I told her the story of our family tree. This time I included Larry in it.

The following week was Easter Sunday. Mollie insisted on keeping a family tradition going. Our sister, Nancy, took us shopping for eggs, dye, and the food she always had for Easter breakfast. Mollie also wanted to go and get flowers for her mother-in-law and Larry's sister Nancy. It was a good day for Mollie. She did what she had to do to keep up her family tradition of Easter breakfast at her house.

Mollie insisted on buying three dozen eggs. I thought OK; she's making salads and maybe pickled eggs for her breakfast. Well, the day before Easter, she directed me to boil the eggs. I said, "One dozen?" "No all three," she replied. "What are we going to do with three dozen hard-boiled eggs?" I asked. "Dye them!" she said. We did with a little help from our sister Nancy's granddaughter, son, and daughter-in-law.

The next day was Easter Sunday. I got Mollie's breakfast started and waited for company. Mollie wasn't having a good day; she would fall asleep in-between bites of her food, and we would have to call her name to wake her up. But she was determined to keep her holiday tradition, including going to her mother–in-law's for the afternoon—which we did. For the most part, Mollie did her best but kept falling asleep sitting in a chair. Her feet and hands were swollen. Larry's sister, Nancy, made a comment to Mollie about her being swollen. Mollie claimed it was from the medicine and her chemo treatments.

I didn't comment on her condition, because I had my own theory about it: it wasn't from chemo or meds. It was her cancer spreading in a deadly force and nothing, not chemo or medicine, was going to stop it. I realized that she was fighting her cancer as she was trying to keep her Easter the same as it was while Larry was alive. These thoughts I kept to myself as I went into the kitchen to sit with Larry's Mom and Dad.

Larry's Dad was so sad and quiet as he looked out the kitchen window. His Mom, well, she was a feisty ole soul. She kept up with the smiles and the laughter of how all her flowers were yellow, and how she would have liked the purple tulips Mollie had bought for Larry's sister Nancy. It wasn't long after being in the kitchen that Mollie soon came in.

She managed to get Larry's Dad to tell me how he and his wife first met. Both of them had musical talents. Both sang for a church group in their younger years, and up until a few months ago, they sang in the church choir. Larry's Dad's health would no longer allow him to walk up the stairs to the church balcony where the choir sang.

Mollie's spirits were lifted as they began to reminisce about Larry and Mollie, and the love they had for him and her. Mollie got through that day. When she went to bed that night, we talked. She told me how happy she was about her Easter breakfast and that she had gone to Larry's mother's house and spent the day with his family. Mollie made it a point to thank me every chance she got for coming to stay with her. She was always so appreciative.

It was during this visit our sister Nancy called to let me know she was coming over to spend the night. I informed

Mollie, and she was so happy referring to it as a "sister pajama party". The three of us sat in the parlor and looked through pictures of days gone by. Mollie went and got a bag that was full of items from when Larry passed away. It contained sympathy cards, Larry's cross and other items from his casket. This was the first time Mollie had looked at these items. She expressed to us how happy she was to finally do it. When it came time to retire for the night, I was placed on the couch while Nancy took over my side of the bed next to Mollie. It was then I decided to throw pillows at her and started a good old fashioned pillow fight. Of course, I lost; both Mollie and Nancy agreed that I should sleep on the couch. Seems that after Larry passed, Nancy stayed with Mollie, and Larry's side of the bed became Nancy's.

As I laid there on the couch, I couldn't help but be thankful for the close relationship Nancy and Mollie had. I always knew Mollie was in good hands with my brothers and sisters, and during this visit, I found it out with all certainty. My brothers would come over and change her furniture around to give the house a different look while a few of my sisters cleaned and dusted. There wasn't a day that would go by when one or more of my family would call or just pop in to see if she needed anything. Yes, our Mollie was very well looked after not only by family but friends as well. Mollie's friends would bring over cooked meals, water—whatever they thought she would need or want. This is when I realized how blessed Mollie and Larry were, not just with family but with friends as well—true friends.

During our quiet times together, Mollie would tell me stories of her visits with Larry while he was in hospice, and how she had asked him if he was afraid to die. He told her, "No, I'm at peace with myself and don't you be afraid either."

She shared with me how she told his parents that if there was anything they wanted to do for their son to go ahead and do it. "I married him," she told them. "But he's yours. You had him." She shared how his mother had kissed her and asked, "What do you want me to do?" Mollie told her, "Go buy him an outfit. You know what he likes to wear. Go do that for your son."

She told me of the time when Larry's brothers were in his hospice room playing musical instruments and singing songs from when they had their own band. If they couldn't remember the lyrics, Larry would tell them. As sick as he was, music was still in his heart as it had been when he and his brothers would get together, and pay tribute to the oldies but goodies.

We began to reminisce about my son Mat's wedding. Larry and our sister-in-law, Marisa, sang to a Meatloaf song. Both were a big hit, especially with the photographer. He kept the video on them for the entire song. I will say both did a good job and put on a good show. Larry was always a good singer and for the first time I thought Marisa had some talent also. I listened to Mollie talk with an aching heart. My eyes full of tears, but at the same time, I tried to give her comfort. My two week visit went by quickly. I was soon off on a plane to California.

I kept in contact with Mollie every day, and my sister Judy about her condition. Mollie was not getting any better. She could no longer take chemo, and it was all a matter of time.

It wasn't long before I received a call from Judy telling me Mollie was being admitted to hospice for pain treatment. Her pain was so high that medication couldn't comfort her. I kept in contact with Mollie while she was there, and I could tell by our conversations, it wouldn't be long. Judy called me again and told me that Dr. McKenna had informed her that Mollie had one to six months to live. I instructed her to call me if anything changed. I promised Mollie I would be there to hold her hand when her time came.

The very next day, I received another call from Judy. "Ger, get on a plane as soon as you can. Mollie has taken a turn and it won't be long." My husband, Howard, got me on a plane on Thursday. My son Eric made frequent phone calls to me and kept telling me, "Mom she may be gone before you get here. I want you to prepare yourself." I told him that she would wait. She won't go without me there. I knew she wouldn't because of our many personal conversations together regarding her feelings of dying, and how she was afraid of the unknown.

When I arrived at the Scranton Wilkes-Barre airport, my daughter-in-law Chrissy was waiting for me. Chrissy married my oldest son Mat on Mother's Day in May of 2008. As I got into her car, the first thing I asked was if Mollie was still with us. "Yes," she said. At that moment my phone rang. It was Eric, "Mom, you're not going to believe this, but Aunt Mollie is very patiently waiting for you. She's sitting up in her bed doing a little dance saying, "Yeah, Gerri's coming." I laughed and said, "I told you she would wait for me."

The airport wasn't far from the Dunmore Hospice center where she was. My stomach felt like a volcano ready to erupt. It was one thing knowing my sister was going to leave us because of cancer, but it was another thing to watch her. Upon my arrival, I was greeted by my son Eric outside the hospice facility. Members of the Naughton and Moraski families were also there waiting to say goodbye to Mollie.

I entered her room which was filled with more members of both families. I walked up to Mollies' bed; she was in the sleeping stage—no longer awake waiting for me. There were no tubes coming from her body and no machines monitoring her. This is what I had envisioned of both her and Larry in a hospice. She was free from all of this and sleeping very peacefully. I began to talk to her knowing she could hear me. "Mollie, do you want me to tell you the story of our family tree?" To my surprise she replied with a quiet "yes" almost as if it took all her energy to speak.

I started my story by reminding her of the first time I told it to her. Larry was lying in bed next to her eating a big piece of chocolate cake (which he shouldn't have been eating since he was diabetic), and how Larry said, "Ger, you do tell beautiful stories. That was nice." I began to tell her the story as I had done many times before, only this time one more person would be added to the tale. I explained how God would come with his arms outstretched to her branch, and how Mom, Dad, and now Larry, would be by his side. While telling her the story, I tried to hold back my tears, but the heartfelt sadness was too great to keep me from crying. I sat by her side holding her hand, waiting for that time to come that deep down inside I wished would just go away. I wanted to be in a nightmare waiting to wake up.

Mollie didn't wake up while we were there, and it was getting late. Family members began to go home except for Judy, Nancy and myself. We were the ones that would sleep in Mollie's room. I watched over Mollie while they tried to get some sleep: one in the recliner, and the other on the couch. I was told that Mollie might try to get herself out of bed thinking she would need to go to the bathroom. My duty was to make sure she didn't. We left the TV on all night with no sound to give us light in the room.

The next day was Friday and Mollie was awake off and on all day. Once in a while, she asked for a drink, and every now and then something to eat. However, she couldn't eat. Drinks were given to her from a dropper by one of my sisters, and then, they would carefully rub her neck so she could swallow. Family members came and went that day. As the day went on and night came, Mollie got worse. Her nurse, Linda, came in every hour to check on her. At around ten o'clock she said, "This is it. Her breathing is shallow, and she has a slow pulse rate. It isn't going to be long."

Family members were called and they returned to the hospice room. Linda told us that her shift was over; she would return on Sunday but wouldn't be seeing us—expecting Mollie to be passed on. Mollie continued to hang on that night, and family members again, with the exception of Judy, Nancy and me, went home.

The next day was Saturday, May 9th, her son Danny's birthday. I knew she would go on that day or the next. Sunday was Mother's Day and our brother Donnie's birthday. No way, I thought, is she leaving us on these days.

Saturday was a cake day for Danny. We all sang happy birthday to him. Mollie tried to join in and had a taste of the icing on his cake. She woke up a few times and at one point, looked at me and said, "Ger, I'm going soon." I sadly replied, "I know honey. It's ok." I sat beside her bed and held her hand. At one point she opened her eyes wide and looked at me. She didn't have to say a word. I knew the questions—and as I looked in her eyes, I answered, "No, Mollie, I don't feel bad. I feel sad because I'm going to miss you, and yes, you will always be my sister, always Larry's wife and always Danny and Robert's mother. None of what you are now while you are here with us is ever going to change. You will always be Our Mollie." She seemed to find comfort in those words and fell back to sleep.

Another time she woke up when family members were in the room and stated, "You all know I'm going to die. We only want you to be happy." "We?" I thought. "She said *we*." Mollie woke up again and said, "I told you I'm coming home, but I don't drive." She repeated these words three different times—each time her voice got louder. As I stood by her bed, Mollie sat up in the bed looked toward the wall and shouted, "I told you, I'm going to die tomorrow." My thoughts began to wander. She's talking to someone as if they were right here in her room. People talk about spirits and the afterlife, but I was never quite sure about it. Is this what Mollie was experiencing? Were there angels calling to her or was it Larry's spirit? I wasn't sure who or what she was talking to. But I knew one thing for sure—she was letting them know very adamantly that she was not going to die today. I knew Mollie's personality, and when she said she was going to do something, she did it: not one minute or one day before.

I was getting my thoughts back when our cousin, Maggie, walked into the room with a large box of Dunkin' Donuts. We sat and visited for awhile and talked about Mollie's outbursts, and at times, we laughed. I went through the box of donuts to find one that was filled with vanilla cream. I talked to myself saying, "Nobody gets the vanilla cream filled ones anymore, just the chocolate ones." Before I knew it, I heard Mollie ask, "Ger, what do you have?" "Donuts. Maggie brought donuts for us to eat." "Can I have one of them?" she asked. I looked at my sister Nancy who was standing by Mollie's bed. Nancy said, "I don't think so." Mollie replied,

"Excuse me. Can I have a donut, please?" Knowing Mollie was upset about not having a donut, I quickly asked her what kind she wanted. Seconds later she fell back to sleep.

On Sunday, Mother's Day, Mollie's nurse Linda could not believe that Mollie was still with us. She asked us, "Is anyone missing that she needs to see?" "No, everyone is here," I replied. Judy asked Linda, "Why can't she get over to the other side?" I joined in the conversation and said, "Because she's afraid!" Linda looked at me and agreed, "She's afraid of the unknown." I began to cry, "She made me promise to be with her and hold her hand because of that fear." Judy said, "Ger do it. I never had that conversation with her. She never spoke to me about it." "I've done that," I replied. "It's not working and seeing her like this is bothering me more than if she passed away. I don't like seeing her like this. I know she's not in pain, because you are making her as pain free and as comfortable as possible. But I can't bear to see her like this." While I was holding her hand, I was praying to God to take her. My older brother Frank-o said, "If we all stay out of the room, maybe it would be easier for her to make the transition." "What, and leave her alone? Someone has to be with her. She's afraid and that's what's keeping her here. She doesn't want to leave the people she loves, because she doesn't want us to feel bad. But she's afraid of the unknown."

It was getting late and family members again began to leave. The three of us stayed to watch over Mollie. Judy and Nancy sat on each side of Mollie's bed. I watched as Judy swabbed her mouth to keep it from getting dry, and how she so gently gave her a drink from the syringe, being sure to help her swallow. Both of them repositioned her head to make her comfortable with a "one, two, three" motion—being careful not to hurt her or make her uncomfortable in any way. I sat and watched as my two sisters—Mollie's caregivers for four years—did all they could to help her in every way possible.

I decided to lie down and watch TV to help me fall asleep. Suddenly, I began to hear someone calling Mollie's name. I looked at the clock. It was midnight. I wondered why on earth they were trying to wake her up. I looked up at the bed and saw that Nancy and Judy were asleep, sitting up in chairs. I soon began to hear a strange sound coming from the head of Mollie's bed, while still hearing her name being called. I thought it was coming from the TV. I walked over to the TV and placed my ear next to it, thinking that this is where the sounds were coming from.

At this moment Nancy woke up and asked, "What are you doing?" I asked her if the TV had sound on. "No, it's only on for the light, so we can see what we're doing." I went back to the couch still hearing Mollie's named being called, and the strange sound from the head of her bed that I couldn't figure out.

I thought, "Maybe it is angels calling her, and she's going to leave us soon. After all it was midnight and Mother's Day was over. And she did adamantly tell someone that she was dying tomorrow." I fell asleep listening to "Mollie, Mollie", and the strange sound coming from the head of her bed.

Monday, I awoke and told my sister Judy about what I had heard. She said, "I was wondering what you were doing by the TV." "Jude," I said, "I don't know what that strange noise was, but I know someone was calling Mollie to come to them."

Nurse Linda entered the room. She, Nancy, and Judy started changing the bed for Mollie and getting her washed up for another day of visitors. During this time, I went out to the foyer of the facility. In the center of it was a beautiful waterfall fountain decorated with plants and flowers. I watched as family members were in the kitchen patiently waiting to go in and visit Mollie. I looked around and noticed the pictures on the walls, and the nurses tending to their patients. Everything was all done in a peaceful and happy atmosphere—nothing like I envisioned it would be. I had envisioned it to be the house of death: dark and gloomy with an atmosphere of sadness and dismay. It was the complete opposite. People that were dying knew it, and family members did everything they could, along with the nurses, to make their final days as peaceful and comfortable as possible. I remembered speaking to Judy when she had told me Larry was placed in a hospice facility and how she assured me it was a good thing. Not knowing much or anything at all about a hospice, I wasn't convinced of it. In my mind, it was a way of giving up on a dying family member and placing them in a room to die on their own. My first hand experience here with Mollie changed my thinking. I was happy she was placed here, and without telling anyone, I thought it should have been done sooner. Yes, Mollie was dying, however, the hospice team, and its atmosphere, was helping her to live her last days as fully as possible. I believe the hospice gave both Judy and Nancy peace of mind when it came to Mollie's constant care. In a way the hospice became their home as well. The only time they left was if they really had to.

I sat and listened to the waterfall and let my mind wander. I began to remember Mollie as a little girl, and how she was always smiling and laughing. How as a teenager, she loved to play softball, and with her strength and will power she'd hit many a homerun. I recalled the school plays, and how Mollie loved to sing and dance. She tried out for the school play, "The Wiz Is A Wow" (an adaptation of "The Wizard Of Oz"). She was one of the singing and dancing munchkins. When I would visit my mother, Mollie (still living at home with my Mom and younger brothers and sisters.) would be practicing. While she was practicing, she taught my oldest son Mat, who was about four at the time, the song and dance to "If I Only Had A Brain" sung by the scarecrow. She was always very entertaining, and I couldn't help but laugh at her; she was just so cute and talented. I then began to remember her wedding day—what a beautiful bride she was, and that the priest had commented on her beautiful smile.

My mind continued to wander with pleasant thoughts of Mollie. I remembered that a year ago in May my husband Howard and I had come for my older son Mat's wedding. I hadn't seen Mollie in awhile, and at that time, she looked good. The wedding for all of us was a time to remember. There was dancing, laughing, and simply having a good time. The next day, we (my husband Howard, my sons Eric, Stewart and I) went to visit Mollie at her home. Mollie put a gold chain on my wrist which she wanted me to have. Larry had bought it for her for their anniversary. Because of the chemo and different meds, she was too swollen for it to fit her wrist. I was very happy to accept the gift and gave her a big kiss and hug. She began to cry, "I wish you didn't have to go. I know you do, but I just miss you so much." I assured her that we would come to visit again, and that I would call her often. With these remembrances, my mind gradually drifted back to reality. The peace and serenity of the waterfall gave me a few minutes of comfort before I returned to Mollie's room.

A few of us were in the room when my older brother Frank-o came in asking me to have everyone leave the room so he could be alone with Mollie. I politely asked everyone to leave and asked my brother how long. "I'll let you know when I'm done," he said. As I left the room, I thought, "I pray she goes while he's in there alone with her. Maybe this is what she needs—the strength of our older brother holding her hand, making her feel safe and unafraid." I sat in the kitchen with other family members reminiscing about Mollie and Larry: retelling the stories of their haunted house and laughing because the kids where too scared to go in. I told everyone about my visits, and how Larry took very good care of my sister. Of course, we all laughed when I told the story of the hamper, and how I thought Mollie was going to throw up. Most of my reminiscing was of how I admired the way each one took care of the other. Mollie would think of Larry first, and Larry would think of Mollie first. The two of them had a unique relationship with each other. Did they have their spats? I'm sure they did. I don't believe anyone has a perfect relationship, but I know one thing; they definitely had the perfect love for one another. At least that's the way I saw it with every visit that I had with them. After about fifteen minutes of reminiscing, I decided to go outside for some fresh air. It wasn't long after that when Nurse Linda came to the door and motioned for me to come in. As I walked through the door, she told me, "Mollie's gone. You may go in to see her." As I walked down the hall, my brother Frank-o was walking toward me with tears in his eyes. We gave each other a hug, and I thanked him for staying with Mollie. "She's at peace now with Mom, Dad, and Larry—as it should be." I cried. We all went into the room to say our goodbyes. I gave Mollie a kiss on the cheek and said, "I'll see you again Baby Sister—when my time comes."

Judy and her husband, Bob, made all the arrangements for Mollie: choosing the casket and setting up funeral arrangements. Thursday would be the day of the viewing, and Friday would be her funeral.

On Friday everyone met at the funeral home to say our final goodbyes. After the mortician said his prayers, I walked up to Mollie's casket, gave her a kiss on the cheek, and told her I loved her. I stood for a moment to take one last look at her. I thought about how her body was there, but she wasn't. It was at that moment, I realized we are not bodies with souls, but souls with bodies. Mollie's soul had left the body it had occupied and went into the transition of another world with so many other loved ones that had passed on. I began to read the story of "Our Family Tree", which I told her many times during her illness. However, this was the first time she would hear it in the form of a poem.

OUR FAMILY TREE

Years ago our parents, Francis Naughton
and Josephine Magnone,

were united in marriage and planted their family tree.

Each branch was different in shape and size.

They all grew and flourished as they reached for the skies.

One branch, the baby girl, had the most beautiful smile.

She became ill as she stretched her rugged mile.

She struggled and fought the most courageous fight.

As all the other branches loved and held her tight.

God had other plans for this branch on our tree.

He decided it was time for a rest for our Mollie B.

He came with his arms stretched out to her branch.

With Mom, Dad and Larry beside him,
they motioned with a glance

For Mollie to come, for their baby needed a rest.

While Larry whispered softly, "Come
Mollie. We're God's special guest."

She spread her wings as she began to take flight.

Turned with a smile to let the other
branches know she'd be all right.

She took their hands as their wings spread wide.

She found her place with Mom, Dad,
and Larry next to God's side.

Her branch though wilted on our tree it will stay.

For I cannot and will not say Our Mollie
is dead—she is just gone away.

When I finished reading Mollie's poem, it was time to leave for the church. As I sat in a pew next to my sister Judy, I heard the organ begin to play. Goose bumps engulfed my body as I grabbed Judy's hand. "Judy!" I whispered. "That's it. That's the noise I heard in Mollie's room while someone was calling her name!" Judy looked at me with astonishment and surprise. This is when I knew for certain our sister Mollie was in the hands of God and his angels, along with our parents, and her soul-mate Larry. I knew at that moment that she would definitely be okay. Our niece Bryne read her eulogy; she spoke not only of Mollie but of Larry, and the love they had for each other. She spoke of their struggles with cancer, and how, when she was a little girl, both she and her sister were petrified to go into their much famous haunted house. She spoke of how our sisters, Judy and Nancy, did the tag teaming when taking care of Mollie, and the love and support Mollie had from family and friends throughout her illness. She spoke of Mollie's love of the children she cared for at St. Joseph's Center. Bryne did a beautiful job on Mollie's eulogy, and it was proper and fitting to include Larry in it.

After the funeral, we went to a restaurant to have brunch. For the second time in less than two months, the Naughton and Moraski families were united together for the passing of a family member. First was Larry, a member of the Moraski family and second, Mollie, a member of the Naughton family. I wasn't there in body when Larry passed. However, I was definitely there in spirit. I could sense the sadness in Larry's parents as we sat for brunch. Larry's Mom, at one point, made a remark to me on how she just buried her son, and now she was losing a daughter. That's how they felt and thought of Mollie: not as a daughter-in-law but as a daughter. The funny part of it all was I knew how they felt. Larry, to me, was more than a brother–in-law—he was family.

After the brunch was over, I let everyone know I was going back home to California first thing in the morning. I gave everyone my love and said my goodbyes. While at home sitting in our parlor with my husband Howard, he looked at me and said, "He gave her the perfect gift." "Who?" I asked. "Larry, he gave your sister the perfect gift." It was then I saw that he was looking at the screen-saver on our computer. It was a picture of Mollie and Larry in their kitchen which I had taken of them on my Christmas visit. It was the last time I saw Larry. And I remembered how he knew he had cancer and chose not to do anything about it, because if he did, he wouldn't be able to take care of Mollie. I looked at my husband and said, "You're right. He did give her the perfect gift. He gave her the gift of love."

Mollie and Larry didn't live among the rich and famous. Their lives were simple. They worked hard for what they had, and both were proud of their achievements. My sister Mollie, after the passing of her husband, gave me permission to write this book, and I know she would be happy to invite you to visit their world through pictured memories.

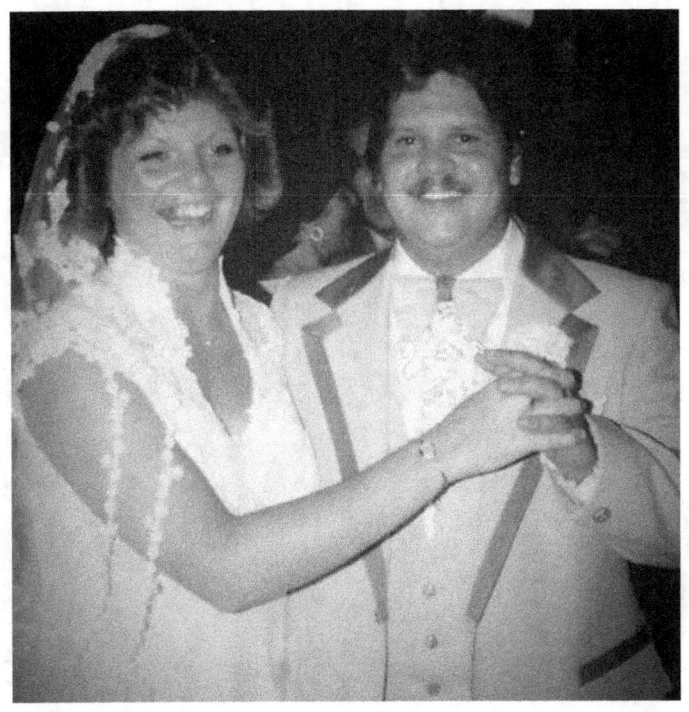

Mollie and Larry united in marriage on July 5, 1980 and formed a love so strong that cancer itself could not come between them.

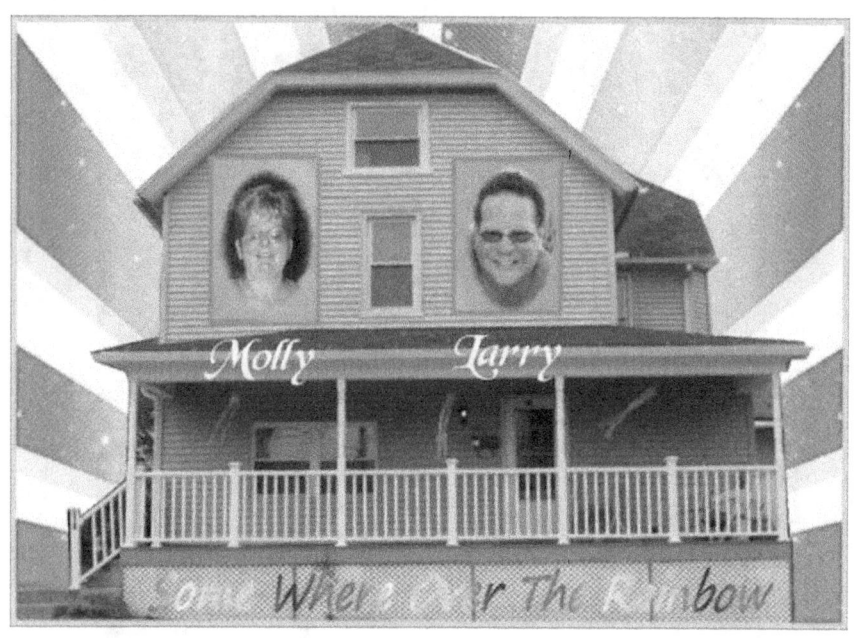

Mollie and Larry's home established on July 5, 1980.

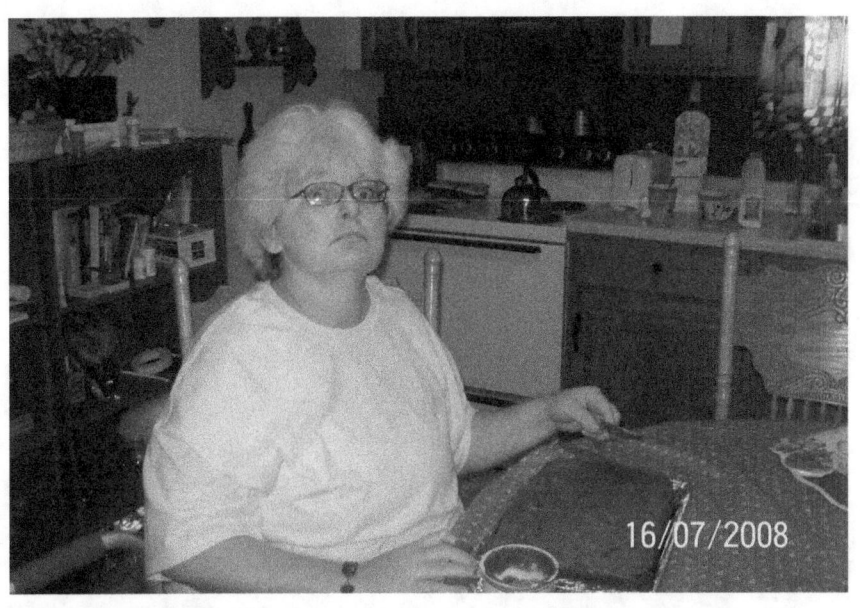

Mollie decorating Larry's birthday cake.

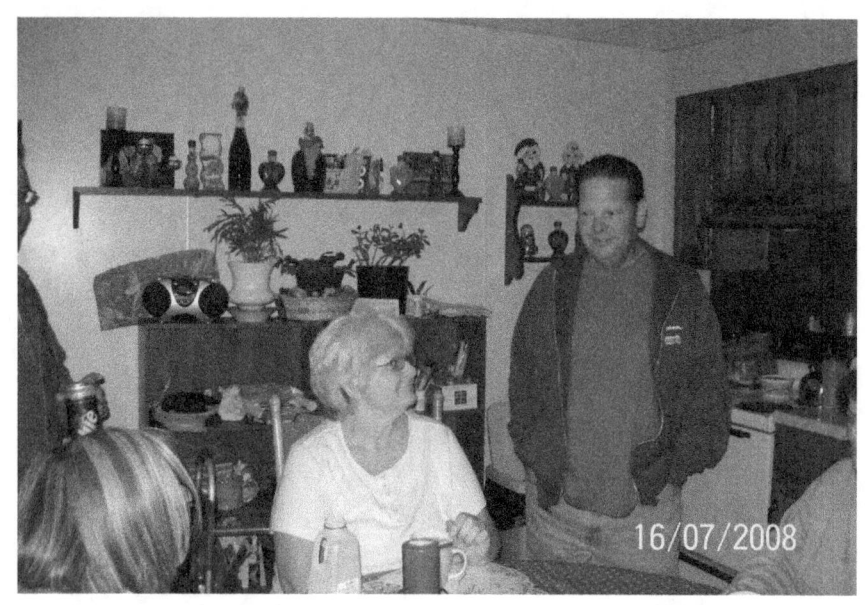

Mollie and Larry after we sang Happy
Birthday to him and enjoyed his cake.

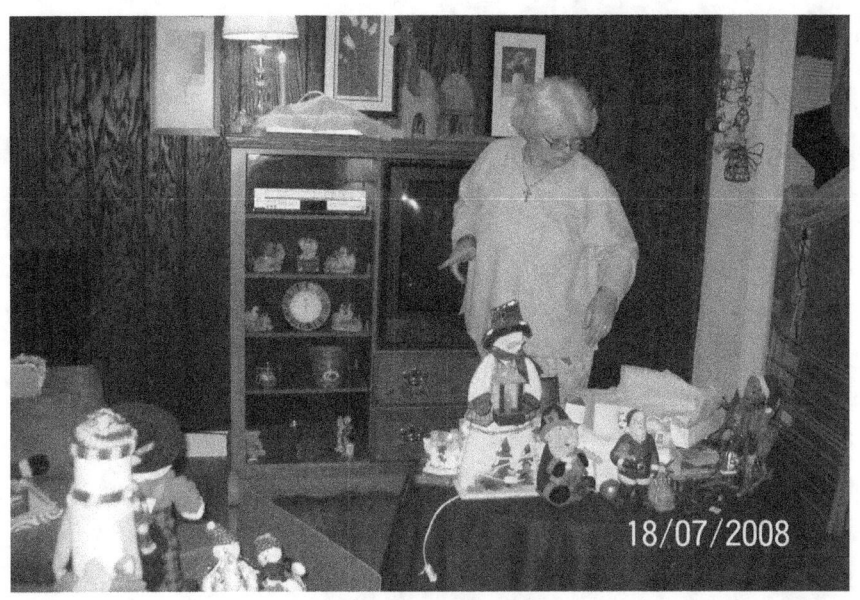

18/07/2008

Mollie on one of her better days decorating for Christmas.

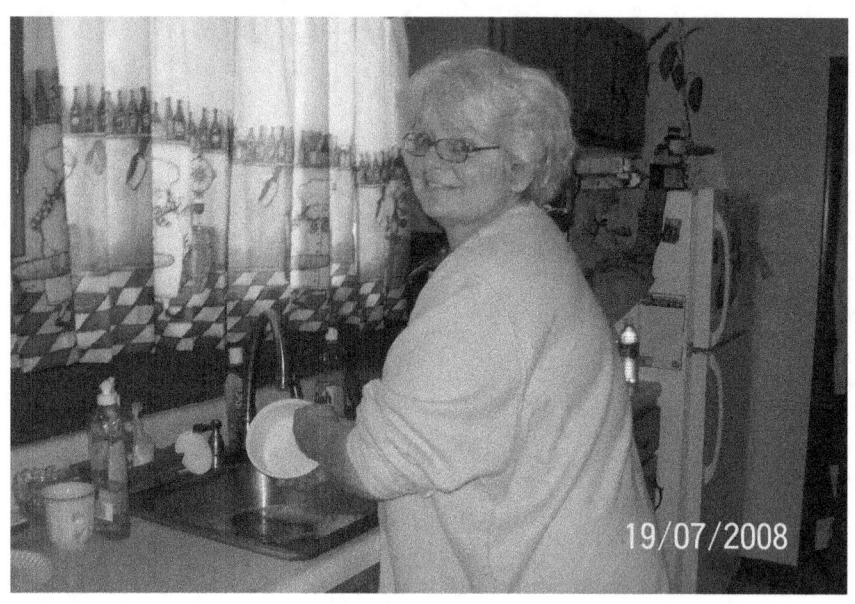

19/07/2008

I love this picture! This was a day she had so much energy she decided to wash the dishes, and I would dry them. I told her she reminded me of Mrs. Claus.

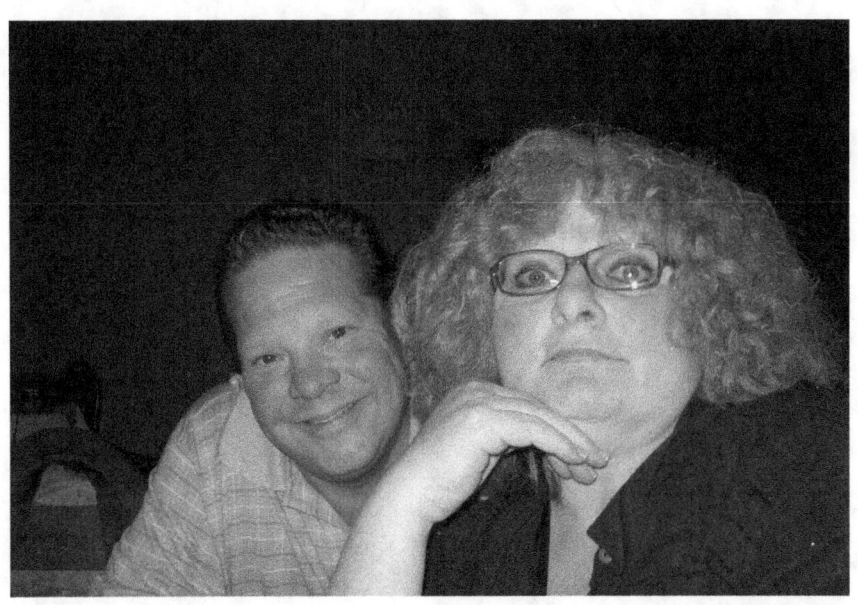

Mollie and Larry enjoying my son Mat's wedding,
May 11, 2007.

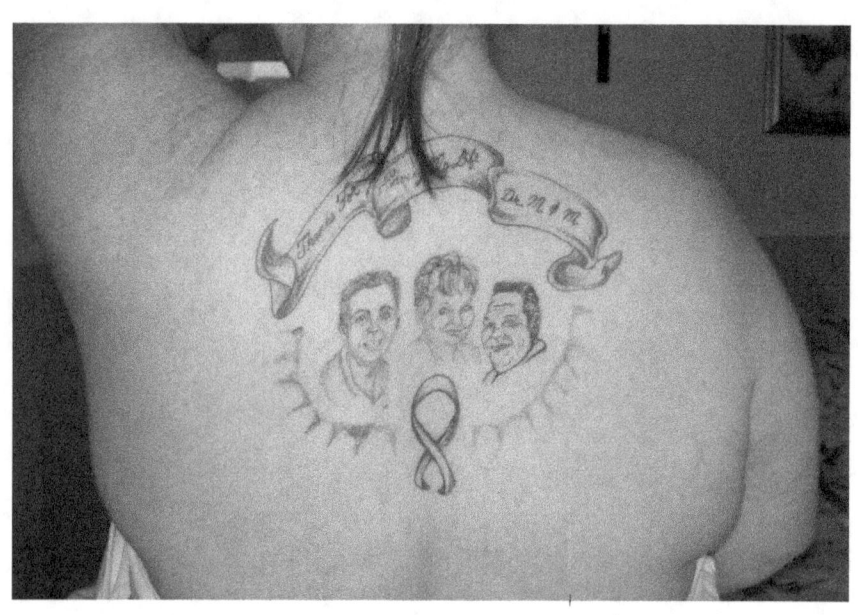

Mollie's famous tattoo of her Doctor, Larry and her.
"Thanks For Saving My Life"

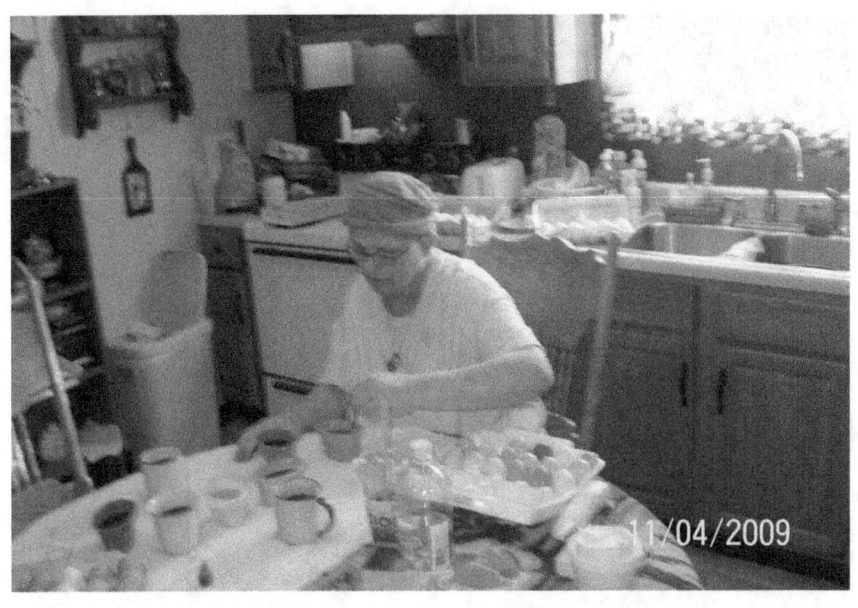

Mollie dying eggs for the Easter Bunny.

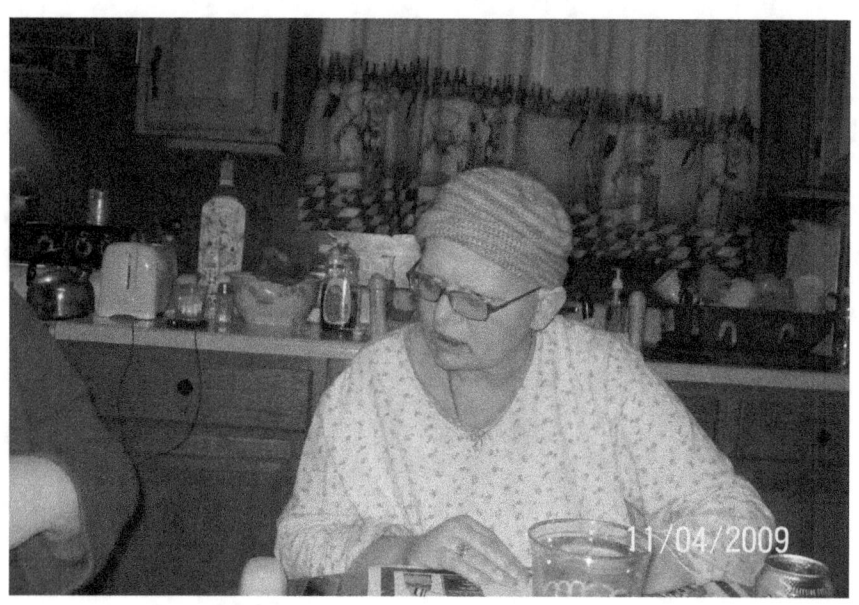

Easter breakfast: she had a very hard day and still managed to get dressed and go visiting her in-laws so she could keep up her family tradition.

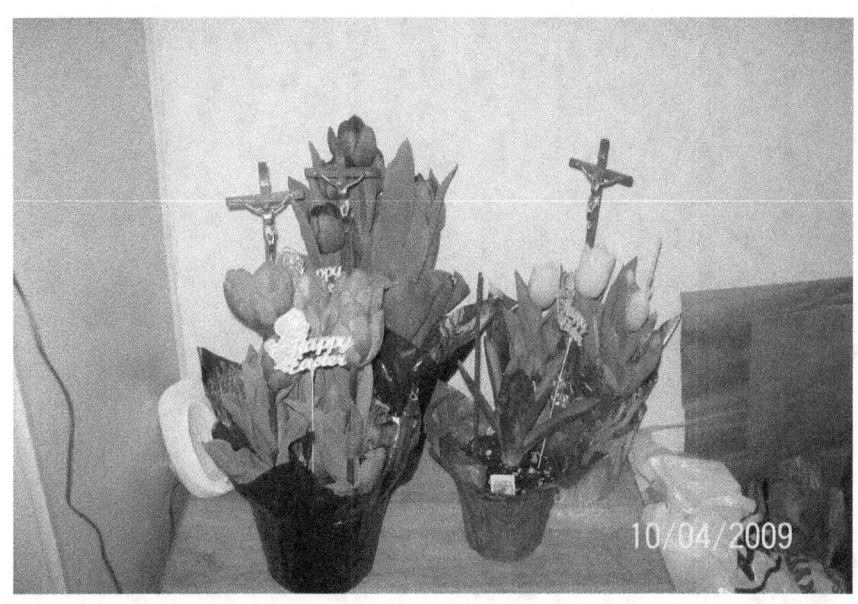

My sister Nancy took us shopping so Mollie could
pick out Easter flowers for her family.
She did a very good job and got some nice colored ones.

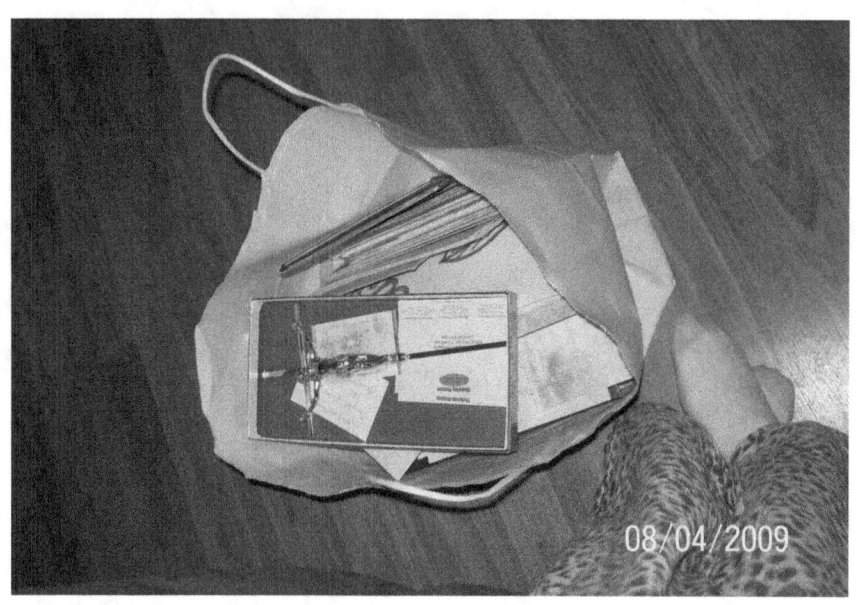

In this bag were Larry's items from his coffin, and sympathy cards. She finally got to look at them the night we had the sleep over with Nancy.

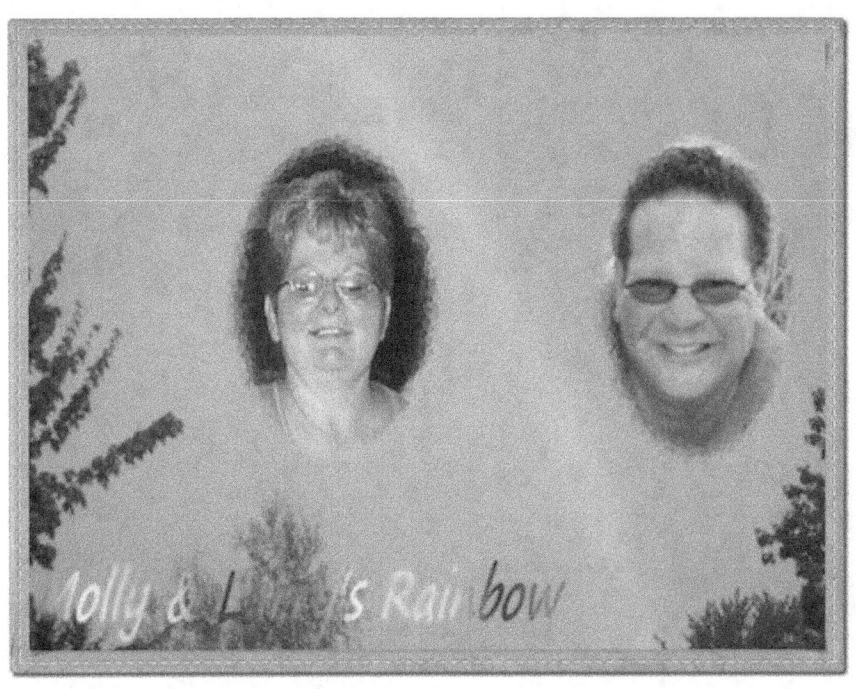

Somewhere over the rainbow when our
time comes, we will meet again.

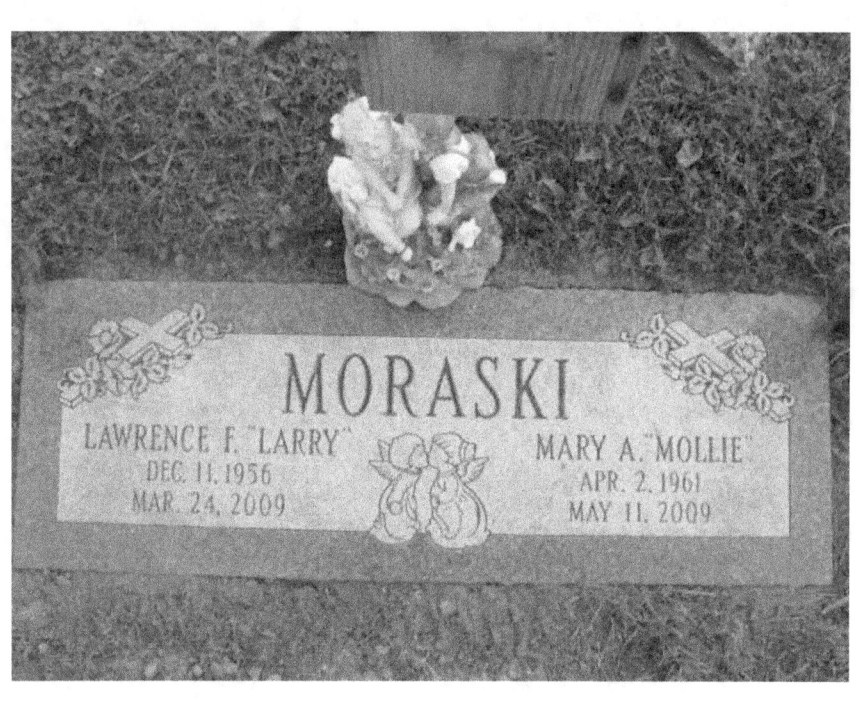

MORASKI

LAWRENCE F. "LARRY"
DEC. 11, 1956
MAR. 24, 2009

MARY A. "MOLLIE"
APR. 2, 1961
MAY 11, 2009

The Peaceful Path

I walked a peaceful path today.

I saw different folks along the way.

The sky was blue, the sun quite bright.

The air was fresh to my delight.

Through the path I strolled as my thoughts wandered.

How peaceful this path—here and yonder.

The folks I saw didn't speak a word:

Elderly, young, and babies-not a word.

Taking the path up a small hill,

I noticed a white lamb that sat very still.

He didn't move nor make a sound.

He sat so peaceful as if no one was around.

I happened upon a Mom and Dad

With two young girls, and I became sad.

My heartfelt heavy as I held back my tears.

The dates were the same including the years.

I couldn't help wonder what happened that day.

I knew in my heart—God had the final say.

This peaceful path and all of its quest

Was the final place of their eternal rest.

I strolled down the path with a grace and stride.

Knowing all who rested here were God's chosen pride.

www.ingramcontent.com/pod-product-compliance
Lightning Source LLC
Chambersburg PA
CBHW060650290526
45793CB00001B/475